In Defense of the Life of the Unborn

by
Jesús A. Diez Canseco

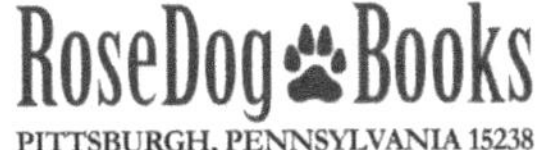

RoseDog Books
PITTSBURGH, PENNSYLVANIA 15238

The contents of this work, including, but not limited to, the accuracy of events, people, and places depicted; opinions expressed; permission to use previously published materials included; and any advice given or actions advocated are solely the responsibility of the author who assumes all liability for said work against any claims stemming for the publication of the work.

All Rights Reserved
Copyright © 2022 by Jesús A. Diez Canseco

No part of this book may be reproduced or transmitted, downloaded, distributed, reverse engineered, or stored in or introduced into any information storage and retrieval system, in any form or by any means, including photocopying and recording, whether electronic or mechanical, now known or hereinafter invented without permission in writing from the author.

RoseDog Books
585 Alpha Drive, Suite 103
Pittsburgh, PA 15238
Visit our website at www.rosedogbookstore.com

ISBN: 979-8-88729-059-1
eISBN: 979-8-88729-559-6

DEDICATION

Dedicated to the principle that life begins at conception and must be protected and defended until natural death.

TABLE OF CONTENTS

INTRODUCTION

Throughout the history of humankind, the right to life of unborn humans was, for the most part, protected by every human community. The justification of that right was based on the fact that an unborn human being has no other source of protection than that provided by his parents or the collectivity in which they lived. The first human communities welcome the birth of new people inasmuch as they were vital to the survival and progress of the community itself.

The world's first legal codifications, such as those enacted by the Mesopotamians and the Egyptians, prohibited any practice which could cause a premature ending to the mother's pregnancy or the killing of the newly born children. The Greek and Roman civilizations continued the legal precedents inasmuch as they contributed to benefit the slave economic mode of production prevalent at that time. For instance, a woman in child-bearing age was, usually, more expensive because she could give birth to future productive slaves. During the Middle Age, Roman Law included stipulations granting civil rights to the unborn child provided he was born alive.

The existence of antiabortion legal norms become all the more necessary as a means to restrain the proliferation of abortion practices motivated by the reduction of the number of weaker children, the intent to hide sexual activity, the killing of physically-disfigured newborn children, the elimination of unwanted heirs, the need to avoid the expenses and burdens of child-rearing, and so forth.

In contemporary times, with the globalization of the means of mass communication, the issue relating to the right to life of the unborn human beings has fallen into the realm of the public domain. There is much controversy, vitriolic debate and even violence between two radically polarized groups: Pro-choice and Pro-life.

On June 24, 2022, the U.S Supreme Court ruled that the Constitution does not confer a right to abortion, thus overturning the decision known as Roe v. Wade, which, for almost 50 years, had legalized abortion. Nevertheless, the confrontation between pro-abortion and anti-abortion groups continues to permeate the political, religious, economic, scientific, technological, and other institutions of society.

This book presents, in a brief and concise manner, a series of thoughts in defense of the right to life of the unborn human.

The Author

CHAPTER I

HUMAN LIFE BEGINS AT CONCEPTION

HUMAN LIFE AT THE BEGINNING

At the very time of conception, the newly conceived human being contains in himself all the essential elements of his individual human life. After that, all he needs to do is to develop them.

––––––––––

HUMAN DEVELOPMENT

The developmental progress achieved by the unborn human being from the time of conception until the time of his birth is as marvelous as the progress he achieves from the time of his birth until the time of his natural death.

––––––––––

NOT AN ACT OF MAGIC

To deny that life begins at conception is the equivalent to saying that the birth of a child is an act of magic – like when a magician pulls out grown rabbits out of his hat.

––––––––––

PRIORITIES ARE PRIORITIES

How can man attempt to learn about the beginnings of the universe, if he has not yet learned that his own life begins at the time of his conception?

———————

AGE DOESN'T MATTER

If we agree that the condition of being human has nothing to do with age, then, we have to agree that a newly conceived child is as much a human as a newly born child.

———————

THE PROCESS OF MATURATION

If we state that a human being, who has been for two weeks in his mother's womb, is not human because he has not reached maturity, the question arises, when does a human being reach maturity? It is a solid biological principle that the process of maturation for living beings is a lifelong process.

———————

SIMILARITIES

In many ways, society is an organism that resembles the organism of an individual human being. For instance, when a woman resorts to abortion in order to preserve the beauty of her body, she resembles a society that resorts to eliminate the disabled in order to preserve the purity of the race.

———————

FIGURING OUT OUR LIFE EXPECTANCY

In figuring out our life expectancy, we must include the time we spend in our mother's womb.

AGE

At the time of his birth, a child is already nine months old.

RACE AND AGE

Racism discriminates between people's races. Abortion discriminates between people's ages.

THE NOBILITY OF THE HUMAN RACE

Any attempt to make the human race nobler by eliminating the unborn child will only degrade human beings to a level below that of any animal species. The nobility of the human race is solely founded on the respect for life at any stage.

A MANIFESTATION OF ART

The entire life of a human being is a beautiful manifestation of art, and its most magnificent revelation happens at the time of conception.

ESSENTIALLY EQUAL

Physiologically, the differences between man and woman are numerous; but, when it comes to the function of procreation, man and woman are absolutely equal, for it is impossible for procreation to occur without one or the other.

SHAMEFUL ALLIANCE

The goal of a pro-life movement is to promote life; therefore, it cannot be allied to any movement that promotes war.

———————————

INTENSIVE NURTURING

The future of humanity receives nine months of intensive nurturing in a mother's womb.

———————————

THE BEAUTY OF LIFE

The true art lover is someone who appreciates and enjoys the beauty of human life in all its stages from conception to natural death.

———————————

CLOSE TO IMMORTALITY

Through love and procreation, man gets as close to immortality as he possibly can get in his mortal life. Through love, he not only procreates but also cares for the child throughout his entire life. The child, therefore, becomes sort of the first installment towards an immortal succession of new human beings.

———————————

EXACTLY THE SAME

Nature has determined that maternity and paternity are exactly the same, except for the cycle of pregnancy.

———————————

UNITY: THE BEGINNING AND THE END

Unity has always been the origin and the final destiny of human beings. In his origin a human being is the product of the unity of the female egg with the male spermatozoon. And, his final destiny is the return to the unity of heaven and earth.

CREATION AND EVOLUTION

A process of evolution follows every act of creation; and the conception of a human being is not an exception.

GETTING READY

It takes several years for a child to become ready to move out of his home and into the world. It takes about nine months for an unborn child to become ready to move out of his mother's womb and into the world.

CONSISTENCY

When somebody says he loves humanity but does not love the unborn children, is a liar because there are no human beings who have not spent the first months of their lives in the womb of a mother.

WHO FEELS THE PAIN?

Abortion may cause no pain to the mother or to the abortionist, but it certainly causes much pain to those who love human life.

EYES CLOSED

He who closes his eyes in the face of abortion might as well close them in the face of one of humanity's greatest holocausts.

HE ONLY WANTS TO LIVE

Since the moment of his conception, the unborn child wants to live. If that were not the case, no unborn child would be able to complete his development in his mother's womb.

I TAKE OFFENSE

It is offensive to me to hear some people say that I was not a human being when I was in my mother's womb.

A MEMBER OF A COMMUNITY

Since the moment of his conception, the child is an active member of a community – the community he establishes with his mother.

WE'VE GOT THE INVITATION

By virtue of having been conceived in our mother's womb, we have received an invitation to attend the banquet of life.

BEYOND UNFITNESS

When the parents fail to provide for the needs of their newly born child, we call them unfit parents. What can we say of the parents who decide to abort their newly conceived child?

WHAT A BAD IDEA!

To the abortionist, conceiving a child is like conceiving a bad idea: you may remove the newly conceived child from the womb of his mother, just as a bad idea can be removed from someone's head.

EXPECTATIONS OF A PREGNANT MOTHER

Upon learning that she is pregnant, a woman who knows the value of human life will say to her friends, "I am expecting a child". Would the pregnant woman, who intends to have an abortion, say to her friends, "I am expecting a nonhuman?"

ALREADY A MOTHER

A woman who says she wants to have an abortion because she doesn't want to be a mother, forgets she is already a mother.

MAKING LIFE SHORT

There must be something terribly wrong in a society where the interval between the beginning and the end of life is set to last approximately 20 years, as in the case of war, or no more than a few months, as in the case of abortion.

WORST ENEMIES

Abortion and artificial means of contraception are the worst enemies of human development.

HE WAS WRONG

At the time of his conception, the unborn child is convinced that his parents know what they are doing; abortion proves him wrong.

HIDDEN REASON

When measuring the life expectancy of human beings, the statistician prefers not to include the deaths caused by abortion for the simple reason that it would significantly lower the average number of years the average person lives.

———————

RESPONSIBLE PARENTS

Responsible parents would do everything in their power to protect the life of their newly born child. Similarly, responsible parents would do likewise to protect the life of their newly conceived child.

———————

MALIGNANT AND BENIGN TUMORS

The abortionist claims that abortion is necessary for some women, but not for others. For the women in the first group, the unborn child is like a malignant tumor that must be removed. For the women in the second group, the unborn child is a benign tumor that does not need to be removed. In any case, the mother will be cured of the tumor by the end of nine months. Is the abortionist talking about a miraculous cure?

———————

GIFTS

Life is a gift from God to man; respect for life is man's gift to God.

———————

WHY

The newly conceived human being does not know why he is alive; many of his adult brothers don't know why either.

———————

NOT A CHRONOLOGICAL CATEGORY

One month in our mother's womb is, approximately, the equivalent to ten years outside her womb. But since human life cannot be reduced to a mere chronological category, we must give equal respect to those who are expecting to be born and those who have already been born.

ANSWERS HE CAN LIVE WITH

At the time of his conception, the unborn child presents us with many questions. It is our responsibility to give him answers he can live with.

HUMAN EQUALITY

At the time of conception, every person is the living proof of human equality. We all were humanly equal at that young age, and we will continue to be humanly equal at any other age.

CHANGING

Since the time of conception, the unborn child and his mother are two distinct human beings, changing in different ways. In the first nine months, the changes experienced by the mother are insignificant in comparison with the changes experienced by the newly conceived child.

BOTH ARE HUMAN

The one-month-old child shown on the ultrasound computer screen does not look like a human being; neither does the one-year-old, skin-and-bones child shown on the TV's evening news. Believe me, they are both human beings!

ACCURACY

It is not accurate to say: "Those who are born will die someday". It is accurate: "Those who are conceived will die someday". Death is death whether it happens when we are in our mother's womb or when we are one hundred years old.

———————

ASHAMED OF HIMSELF

He who promotes abortion is ashamed of his humble formation in the womb of his mother.

———————

PROTAGONISTS

The first truth about the unborn child is that his conception is the product of the union between his mother and father. And the first lie is abortion. We adults are protagonist and witnesses of the truth and the lie.

———————

TWO GREAT MYSTERIES

For those who are still in the world, life after death is a great mystery. For those who are still in their mother's womb, life after birth is a great mystery.

———————

LOGICAL CONCLUSION

If the newly conceived child is not a member of humanity, then humanity is exempt from the evolution of life.

———————

A WORLD WITHOUT BEGINNINGS

To live in the world without loving the unborn is like living in a world without beginnings.

———

DEMONSTRATION OF LOVE

A pregnant mother demonstrates love when she wishes the best for herself as well as for her unborn child.

———

CONTRACEPTIVES

Contraceptives are instruments against the right to be conceived.

———

LETHAL PROPORTIONALITY

In order to kill a strong man, a killer uses a gun. In order to kill a newly conceived child, the mother swallows a morning-after pill.

———

PSEUDOSCIENCE

Pseudoscience arrives at conclusions based only on external appearances. When a scientist arrives at the conclusion that the newly conceived children are not a human being, he is a pseudoscientist.

———

AN ABSURD BELIEF

Those who believe that the unborn child is not a human being until the moment of his birth, must believe that the first breath of air the child takes into his lungs is the all-powerful creator of life.

———

A DIFFERENCE

The difference between the unborn human beings and those who have already been born is that life is not optional for those in the first group.

NO DIFFERENCE AT ALL

During his life in his mother's womb, the unborn child grows with the help of his mother. During his life outside his mother's womb, he continues to grow with the help of his mother.

COMMON DENOMINATOR

All the good deeds humanity has done have one common denominator – respect for life.

WHAT ELSE COULD HE BE?

The undeniable proof that the unborn child is a human being since the moment of his conception is that he continues to be a human being at the time of his birth.

SPEAKING UP

Just like a mother speaks up for the rights of her one-month-old child, she should speak up for the rights of her newly conceived child.

THE GREATEST OFFENSE

The greatest offense a human being can suffer is to be labeled unwanted, especially when he is in his mother's womb.

PRACTICING PATIENCE

Since the time of his conception, the unborn child begins to practice one of the most precious human virtues: patience.

____

GOOD USE OF AUTHORITY

The pregnant mother knows that she is in authority over the child in her womb. She also knows she must use her authority to protect the life of her child.

____

THE MORNING-AFTER PILL

A man and a woman have no control over their bodies when they conceive a child whom they have to kill the morning after.

____

NO CONTROL AT ALL

When a woman exercises control over her body by killing the child in her womb, she is demonstrating that she had no control over her body when she conceived her child.

____

LEFT OUT

If we say that procreation does not occur at the time of conception but at some later time, then we must conclude that the male has no role in procreation.

____

PRODUCT OF MAGIC

I wonder if the abortionist believes he became a human being at the time of his conception. If he does not, then he is the product of an act of magic.

____

A NEW FORM OF LIFE?

If we were to assume, just for a moment, that the newly conceived child is not a human being, then we would have to ask the following question: Who is the creature growing inside his mother's womb? And there are only two possible answers, the child is either a new form of life never before identified, or he is human life in its inception.

TO CHANGE THE WORLD

If a man and a woman believe the world is not appropriate for raising a child, then they have no other choice but to change the world.

TO SEE IT TO BELIEVE IT

Those who believe that the unborn child is not a human being will not change their minds until they see, with their own eyes, that the immediate result of conception is a fully developed person.

EXPLANATIONS ABOUT THE SOUL

The explanation, which leads us to understand that from matter, man evolved into a being with a soul, is the same explanation that leads us to understand that from the moment of conception, a human begins to enrich his soul.

MORE MIRACLES

A human being experiences more miracles in the time between his conception and his birth than in the time between his birth and his death.

ENDURING HAPPINESS

Throughout his entire life, there is no greater happiness for a man than the one he felt when his mother decided not to abort him.

––––––––––

JOY DESTROYED

The unborn child's joy for having being conceived is destroyed only by abortion.

––––––––––

UNITY OUT OF DIFFERENCES

It is a human attribute to bring about unity out of our individual differences, including the individual differences between born and unborn children.

––––––––––

LIFE MUST GO FORWARD

Just as the newly born child cannot go back to his mother's womb, neither can the newly conceived child go back to his father's spermatozoon and his mother's ovum. Life must go forward.

––––––––––

TWO RIGHTS ARE TAKEN AWAY

Abortion takes away the right to be born; contraceptives take away the right to be conceived.

––––––––––

THE DOOR TO ETERNITY

Death is not the door to eternity, conception is.

––––––––––

ONLY ONE NAME

In order to differentiate his various stages of development, man calls himself zygote, embryo, fetus, infant, youth, adult, and elder. Nature just calls him human.

SEQUENTIAL ORDER

It is only a matter of time for the newly conceived human being to be born and to die. It is a sign of wisdom to respect the sequential order of life.

OUR DEVELOPMENT

The proof that the unborn child is a human being lies in his ability to develop from a fertilized egg into a newly born person. Our inability to comprehend such development negatively impacts our development as adult persons.

DEPRIVATION OF LIFE

Abortion means deprivation of life on two counts. First, by preventing the newly conceived child from living in his mother's womb for the number of months he needs to be born; and, secondly, by preventing the unborn child from living in the world for the number of years he needs to make our world better.

THE FIRST HUMAN RIGHT

The first right of a human being, even before his right to be born, is his right to be conceived.

FULL LIFE

Living a full life includes the time we spent in our mother's womb.

LOVE FROM THE TIME OF CONCEPTION

In order to strengthen the bond between a pregnant mother and her unborn child, she must love him from the time of conception.

A COMMON OMISSION

Most biographies omit the most important part of a person's life: the time he spent in his mother's womb.

HONORABILITY

The newly conceived child confers honorability to human conception; his parents share in that honorability after conception.

THREE MUST BECOME ONE

The parents and their newly conceived child are so different from each other that they are presented with the superb challenge to become one family.

A ONE-MILLION-DOLLAR TRANSACTION

Abortion would be unheard of if the conception of a child were not the result of sexual intercourse but instead the result of a one-million-dollar transaction between mother and father.

THE BIRTH OF PARENTHOOD

A man and a woman become parents at the moment they conceive a child; in other words, parenthood is born when a child is conceived.

A RIGHT TO EXPECT

As parents have a right to sexual intercourse, so does a child have a right to be conceived. If the objection to the latter is that he who does not exist, cannot have any rights, then we must conclude that future generations have no right to expect from the present generation a world where they can live.

LIFE IS WORTH LIVING

Every person has the responsibility to demonstrate to the newly conceived child that life is worth living.

"MAKING LOVE" AND "MAKING BABIES"

When abortion is an option, a man and a woman tend to fall into the stupidity of forgetting that "making love" can result in "making babies".

PROTECTION OF LIFE

All advocates for the protection of human life are doomed if they do not advocate for the protection of the life of the unborn first.

TO WELCOME AND TO REJECT

The morning-after pill proves to the newly conceived child that his parents welcome sexual pleasure but reject him.

DOUBLE DEATH

Parenthood begins at conception. To plan the abortion of a newly conceived child is to plan the death of the child, and of parenthood.

PRIZES

If we were to give a prize to the best achiever ever, we would have to give it to the newly conceived child for the great achievements he accomplishes in only nine months; and another prize to his parents for their support.

A CHRISTIAN BELIEF

Christians believe in Christ since he was conceived in his mother's womb.

CHAPTER II

THE UNBORN CHILD
IS A HUMAN BEING

HUMAN NEEDS

The unborn human being requires the help of his mother in order to meet his developmental needs just as much as a grown-up human being requires the help of his fellow human beings in order to meet his developmental needs. Thus, the needs of the unborn child do not render him a nonhuman.

———————

VOICES OF THE FUTURE

The unborn child and the two-month-old baby need a voice to speak on their behalf, just as much as the poor and the destitute need a voice to speak on their behalf. But while the poor and destitute will show their gratitude by eradicating the old world of poverty and hunger, the unborn and the two-month-old baby will show their gratitude by creating a new world of justice and equality.

———————

THE TIME FOR FREE CHOICE

When it comes to responsible human procreation, the time for mother and father to exercise their right of free choice is before the child is conceived. Once conception occurs, free choice is no longer applicable because now there are three persons instead of two.

———————

THE LIGHT OF DAY AND THE UNBORN CHILD

Just like the light of day advances through the other hemisphere until we see it at dawn, so does the unborn child advance from conception until we see him at birth.

———————

A MATTER OF REMEMBERING

To be honest with you, I don't remember what I did when I was in my mother's womb. So why is it that the unborn child can be killed while in his mother's womb on account of not being able to remember what he does?

———————

NO SAY

There are many groups of people all over the world, especially among the poor, who have no say, whatsoever, in the making of laws which directly affect them. One of those groups is that of the unborn.

———————

COMPENSATION

During the time of gestation, the child can survive without the father, but not without the mother. The father compensates by supporting both mother and child.

———————

BODY LANGUAGE

It is true that the unborn child does not communicate through oral language, but he certainly does communicate thorough body language; and the mother understands it perfectly.

———

NO EXCEPTION

The instinct of survival is common to all human beings, and the unborn child is not the exception.

———

BETRAYAL

While in his mother's womb, the unborn child begins to develop trust in the services of the medical profession. Abortion is the betrayal of that trust.

———

FORGIVENESS

It is not uncommon for a mother to be remorseful after an abortion. Fortunately, the voice of God heals the mother by telling her, "Your child and I have already forgiven you."

———

TWO CELEBRATIONS

It makes little sense for a mother and a father to celebrate the birth of their child if they first did not celebrate the child's conception.

———

THE VALUE OF HUMAN LIFE

The greatness of human life consists in that the value of the life of one single unborn child is the same as the value of the life of the entire humanity.

A GREATER SORROW

The death of a loved one always causes sorrow; and the younger the deceased, the greater the sorrow. Therefore, the death of the youngest of the young, the unborn child, must be a cause of an even greater sorrow.

STRONG BUT DEFENSELESS

Given his developmental age, the unborn child is very strong but defenseless in the face of the abortionist's aggression.

PRODUCTIVITY

No one can say that the unborn child is unproductive. He produces a great deal of joy in his parents and a great deal of expectation in his family.

HE CAN BE SEEN

Medical technology now allows us to see the unborn child on a computer screen. So, how can anybody say that the unborn child is not a human being because he cannot be seen?

SIGHT VS. FEELING

The most convincing proof of someone's presence is not so much the sight, but the feeling. And, for sure, a mother can feel the presence of her unborn child in her womb.

DEPENDENCY

Throughout his life, a human being is socially, psychologically and physically dependent on other human beings, especially when he is in his mother's womb.

———————

LOVE THE UNBORN CHILD

If I said that I do not love the unborn child, how could I ever say that I love those who have already been born?

———————

AN ACT OF TERRORISM

It is hard to imagine the terror an unborn child must feel when the abortionist attacks him. It is even harder to understand why this attack is not called an act of terrorism.

———————

FRIGHTENED TO DEATH

The unborn child is so tender and impressionable that if he were to survive the abortion procedure, he might not be able to survive the fear.

———————

FIGHTING FOR OUR RIGHTS

For several centuries, human beings were denied many rights such as the right to gainful employment, the right to vote, the right to free expression, and so forth. Eventually, social struggle conquered those rights. Nowadays, the unborn human being is denied the right to life. Eventually, the struggle for human survival will reinstate that right.

———————

THE BEST LISTENER

When it comes to listening to Mother Nature, nobody does it better that the unborn child; he comes out of his mother's womb when Mother Nature tells him to do so.

———————

BIRTH CANNOT BE THE CAUSE OF INEQUALITY

It is sad to say that some people consider the birth of a human being to be a cause of inequality. This is the alleged inequality: that the conceived child, who reaches birth, is human, whereas the conceived child, who is about to be born, is not.

———————

NO DIFFERENCE AT ALL

If I were to believe that my human nature is different from that of an unborn child, it will not be long before I come to believe that my human nature is different from that of a ninety-year-old person.

———————

MARVELOUS EMOTIONS

Everybody knows that the unborn child does not communicate through words, but through the emotions he arouses in others. How marvelous are the emotions of a mother when she learns that she is bringing a unique human being to this world! How wonderful are the emotions of humankind at knowing that its survival depends upon the children who are to be born!

———————

A PRAYER OF HOPE

Humanity becomes aware of the need for prayer the moment a pregnant mother begins to consider having an abortion. And it is not at all unlikely that those prayers will fill the unborn child with hope.

A DISPLAY OF COMMITMENT

Under legalized abortion, a pregnant mother may say that she has a right to have an abortion. The world may say, "We cannot afford to feed another mouth". The only one who is seriously committed to life is the unborn child who instinctively makes every effort in his power to be born.

HUMANS AND NON-HUMANS

There may be thousands of men killing each other during nine months of war and we call them humans. But when we have an unborn child peacefully growing for nine months in his mother's womb, we dare to call him a nonhuman.

MUST ENJOY LIFE

If the unborn child were able to find out that he is going to be aborted, he would try to enjoy, to the maximum, whatever time he has left in his mother's womb.

THE RIGHT TO APPEAL

Those who are sentenced to the death penalty, have a right to appeal. But the unborn child, who is sentenced to death by abortion, is denied that right.

ADOPTION

The parents, who decide to have the life of their unborn child terminated through abortion, forget that there are relatives and friends who would be delighted to adopt the child.

THE MOST VIRTUOUS

If humility is the greatest virtue, then the unborn child is the most virtuous of all human beings.

"WHENEVER THERE ARE TWO OR MORE..."

When a pregnant mother feels alone and abandoned, she can always resort to Christ's promise, "Whenever two or more are gathered in my name, I am in their midst". This is a heartfelt expression of love from the unborn child to his mother.

CLASS STRUGGLE

By organizing themselves in labor unions, workers have been able to conquered valuable labor rights. I believe that if the unborn children had the power to organize themselves, they would have attained their most basic right to life by now. But, while the workers struggle against their bosses, it is profoundly saddening that the unborn children have to struggle against their own parents.

MORALLY AND SPIRITUALLY

There is no doubt that the unborn child is morally and spiritually superior to the abortionist. At the moment of the abortion, the child forgives his executioner.

EXAMPLE OF UNITY

The unborn children of the world give the rest of humanity the best example of unity: they all are united in their desire to be born.

—————

BULLYING

The most serious form of bullying is abortion, not only because the aggression is against the most defenseless of all victims, the unborn child, but also because the aggression comes from a powerful perpetrator, the State.

—————

THE JUDICIARY UNDER TRIAL

It is a sign of probity for a judicial system to ensure that no innocent human being is found guilty unless it is proven beyond any reasonable doubt. Then, what can we say of a judicial system that not only finds an innocent unborn child guilty, but also condemns him to death through abortion?

—————

FAIR EXPECTATIONS

A mother expects her child to respect life always. The unborn child expects his mother to respect life for at least nine months.

—————

SELF-SUFFICIENCY

If we were to say that an unborn child is not human because he is not self-sufficient, what could we say about the hundreds of millions of poor men, women and children who are not self-sufficient?

—————

SELFISH CONVENIENCE

A matter of convenience and selfishness: it is less expensive monetarily, and less troublesome, emotionally, to kill a child before he is born than to provide for his support after he is born.

FIRST PRAYER

The first thing an aborted child does when he gets to heaven is to pray that his mother will not have any more abortions.

A FAIR PROPOSAL

"Mommy - said the child from inside his mother's womb – "if you support me for nine months, I will support you for your entire life".

FOR WHOM DOES THE CHILD MOURN?

I believe that the victim of an abortion does not mourn for himself, he mourns for his parents.

MOTHER KNOWS

When a physician tells a pregnant mother that her life would be at risk if she carries through with the pregnancy, he should also tell her that it is not the fault of the unborn child. A mother knows her child does not mean ill to her, and he will understand whatever decision she makes.

TAKEN FOR GRANTED

The unborn child only wants what the rest of us take for granted: LIFE!

WASTED GIFTS

The best gifts society has prepared for the unborn child would be wasted if his mother decides to have an abortion.

———————

A VICTIM OF DOUBLE SEPARATION

Any separation, be it emotional or physical, is painful for any grown-up person. Can you imagine how painful it would be for the unborn child to be the victim of both?

———————

BATTLES

We all have our battles to fight; the unborn child just fights to be born.

———————

EVOLUTION OF THE SOUL

The best proof that the human soul evolves is the unborn child; otherwise, we all would be born without a soul.

———————

A FARCE

If we don't love the unborn child, our love for humanity is a farce.

———————

FROM THE HEART

If a woman, walking along a sidewalk were to see a beggar lying on the ground, silently suffering a heart attack, wouldn't she at least use her cell phone to call 911? Why then, wouldn't a pregnant woman have the heart to listen to her unborn child silently begging to be born?

———————

NO NEED OF PROOF

The unborn child does not need to prove to his mother that he is a human being, she just knows.

DEPENDENT

If it is true the argument that the unborn child is not a human being because he is dependent on his mother for survival, we would have to conclude that none of us is a human being because we all are dependent on others for our survival.

RELIANCE

If the unborn child cannot rely on his parents for his survival, on whom can he rely?

EAVESDROPPING

When a pregnant woman discusses the option of abortion with the abortionist, she must be aware that her unborn child may be hearing that killing is OK.

THE MOST BEAUTIFUL GIFT

During his stay in his mother's womb, the child is lovingly preparing the most beautiful gift humanity will ever receive: himself!

INCOMPLETE

One single aborted child makes humanity incomplete.

EVICTION AND ABORTION

An eviction may throw the renter into the ranks of the homeless. An abortion will, for sure, throw the child into the ranks of the dead.

SILENT PRAYER

Many people pray silently, but nobody does it better than the unborn child.

TO SEE BEAUTY

If we see beauty only in the body and not in the soul, we will never see the beauty of the unborn child, or the beauty of anybody else.

CONSOLATION

The victims of abortion have found their consolation in the following gospel text, "Do not be afraid of those who can kill the body but cannot kill the soul".

TO DO AND TO BE.

It is true that we cannot expect the unborn child to do what grown-ups do; but it is absolutely certain that the unborn child is what grown-ups are.

BREAK UP

Abortion is the breakage of the most intimate union between two human beings: the unborn child and his mother.

TWO IN ONE

Pregnancy is beautiful because it depicts the presence of two human beings in one.

LIVING PROOF

The unborn children do not need to prove they are human beings because those who have already been born are living proof of it.

COMPASSIONATE HEART

The unborn child is in the process of developing his brain, but his heart is more compassionate than that of the abortionist.

DIFFICULTIES SEEING

If men have difficulties seeing their own soul, how could we expect them to see the soul of the unborn child?

TO BE LOVED

One of the most difficult challenges of love is to allow others to love us. In this respect, the unborn child has mastered this challenge: he allows everybody to love him.

FOOT IN MOUTH

Sometimes, adults say things that make them believe that they have "put their feet in their mouth". The unborn child does not make those mistakes.

EXCHANGE OF PRAYERS

The unborn child prays for the physical and mental wellbeing of his mother. The mother prays for her own physical and mental wellbeing so she may never consent to abort her child.

TRIDIMENSIONAL ENVIRONMENTS

The unborn child lives in a tridimensional environment: himself, his mother and God. Once born, our selfish world teaches the child to live in another kind of tridimensional environment: me, myself, and I.

IMMUNITY

Suicide has always been, in one way or another, the result of a sort of insanity, which the unborn child has never suffered.

GREAT COURAGE

It is a sign of great courage for the unborn child to want to be born in a world like ours.

"YOU AND I..."

In times of crisis, when a pregnant mother begins to consider abortion, she needs to hear her unborn child telling her, "Mother, you and I against the world".

ROLE MODEL

A pregnant mother is the first and best role model for her unborn child. She must let him be born.

IT IS MY BODY

A pro-abortion woman says "It is my body". But, what about the unborn child's body, is he a ghost?

A BODY WITH TWO HEARTS?

A woman who wants an abortion says: "It is my body"! Is she talking about a body with two hearts? No, she is talking about two bodies!

A CRY AND A SMILE

Pain is the surest way to know we are alive; otherwise, the obstetrician would not slap the newborn baby on the buttocks.

COMPANIONSHIP

The newly born child already knows the meaning of companionship: he learned it during nine months in the womb of his mother.

MOTHER, SAY NO

Given the medical advances in prenatal care, the unborn child has the lowest rate of mortality; granted, of course, that his mother says no to abortion.

THE GOOD OLD TIMES

Upon birth, the child knows that he has left "the good old times" behind.

VOW OF OBEDIENCE

The unborn child has pledged absolute obedience to his mother. He cannot say no if his mother decides to have an abortion.

———————

DOUBLE STANDARD

We cannot say that the unborn child is not a human being because he is under the absolute control of his mother. Many people in the world are under the absolute control of their oppressors, and we call them human beings.

———————

THE GREATEST FEAR

The mere idea of abortion causes the unborn child to be fearful of his own parents.

———————

IN FAVOR OF THE UNBORN

Because I was once an unborn child, I cannot avoid my responsibility to speak up in favor of the unborn.

———————

FAREWELL AND WELCOME

The birth of a child is one of those events in life when the farewell coincides with the welcome. The newborn child says farewell to his mother's womb while the mother welcomes the child to the outside world.

———————

ONE IS FREE, THE OTHER IS NOT

For the first nine months of his life, the unborn child is free from the arbitrariness of the law, but his mother is not.

———————

BY EXAMPLE

The unborn child demonstrates through his example that it is better to preach with deeds than with words.

TRULY COMPASSIONATE

The unborn child is more compassionate than other human beings; he would never approve abortion.

THERE IS SOMETHING WRONG

There is something wrong when humans can be humane with adults but not with the unborn.

MOTHERLY LOVE

A pregnant woman is so full with anticipation that she is convinced that her unborn child is already a fully experienced human being, while she is still learning how to be a fully experienced mother.

A REASON TO PRAY

I cannot think of any reason why an unborn child may wish to be dead. That is why I pray for all pregnant mothers to respect the wishes of their unborn children.

THE HORRORS OF ABORTION

It is natural for an unborn child, and for all human beings, to die someday. What is not natural is that the unborn child should die at so young an age at the hands of his own parents.

COMPOUND PAIN

In addition to the physical pain of death by abortion, the unborn child suffers the emotional pain of being killed by his own parents.

THE BEST CONTRIBUTOR

No one can deny that the unborn child is a contributor to humanity's wellbeing: he ensures the perpetuation of the human race.

MOTHERHOOD

Between a pregnant woman and her unborn child there is no superiority nor inferiority, there is only motherhood.

BODY AND SOUL

The unborn child, as any other human being, has a body to develop and a soul to protect.

WISDOM

The pregnant mother knows she and her unborn child have equal human rights.

TOTAL SHARING

The unborn child knows a lot about sharing, he shares everything with his mother.

IT IS NEVER TOO EARLY TO START LEARNING

Any difficulties the unborn child may have while in his mother's womb will teach him problem solving skills, except, if his mother decides to abort him.

———————

SHARING NEVER STOPS

It is wonderful that the unborn child shares everything with his mother. Wouldn't it be also wonderful that those who have already been born could continue sharing everything with their fellow human beings?

———————

PARENTS GIVE WHAT THEY ARE

If we believe that the parents are human beings, we have no other choice but to believe that the newly conceived child is also a human being.

———————

A MATTER OF CONSISTENCY

A society that treats adult persons as if they were not human beings shows consistency when treating unborn children as if they were not human beings.

———————

TWO WONDERFUL WORLDS

The miracle of motherhood consists in allowing the unborn child to move from the wonderful world in his mother's womb into a world the child is to make wonderful.

———————

LOVE OF NEIGHBOR

Love of neighbor also includes the unborn.

FRIENDSHIP

If you are not a friend of the unborn, how can you say you are a friend of those who have already been born?

"FORGIVE ME", SAYS THE UNBORN CHILD

Morning sickness is a means used by the unborn child to allow his mother to exercise the virtue of forgiveness.

FEELING

I can feel the joy of the unborn child when his mother decides not to have an abortion.

VESTED INTEREST

The unborn child is truly invested in the wellbeing of his mother because his own wellbeing depends on it.

WASTED EFFORTS

All the efforts the child makes in order to be born will be wasted if his mother decides to have an abortion.

LESSER DEPENDENCY

Among all the human beings, the unborn child has the lesser degree of dependency compared to the rest of us. He depends only on his mother, the rest of us depend on the entire society.

EXPERIENCE IN TEAM WORK

One of the virtues of the unborn child is that he already has experience in teamwork when he is born.

NO TWO ARE EXACTLY ALIKE

Just as there are no two men exactly alike, so too are there no two unborn children exactly alike.

TAKING CARE OF TWO BODIES

A pregnant woman has the responsibility to take care of two bodies, her own and that of her unborn child. Therefore, she cannot take care of her body by eliminating the body of her unborn child.

WEALTH AND WELLBEING

If wealth were to be used for the wellbeing of every human being, there would be no abortion because the unborn children would have their share of wealth.

IT MUST BE SEEN ON TV

In accordance with the standards of modern life, some people will not believe that the unborn child is a human being until they see it on TV.

TODAY FOR YOU, TOMORROW FOR ME

Since an unborn child cannot yet pray for himself, we must pray for him.

A COGNITIVE DIFFERENCE

The cognitive difference between the unborn child and the newly born child is that the former knows his mother very well, whereas, the latter must begin to know her all over again.

"RED TAPE"

Just like an undocumented immigrant is alive but does not yet have a resident's card, an unborn child is alive but does not yet have a birth certificate.

THE RIGHT OF EXPRESSION

A mother knows that the child in her womb has the right of expression because the child's ability to express himself is not limited to speech.

ACHIEVING EQUALITY

There was a time, not long ago, when wives were treated as mere possessions of their husbands. Then later, wives rebelled and won equality of rights with their husbands. When women become pregnant, they must realize that the child in their womb is not their possession, but a human being with equal rights.

NAKEDNESS

Unborn children are the image of Adam and Eve in the Garden of Eden: they are naked.

TOO PROUD TO ACCEPT IT

Those who advocate for abortion cannot accept the fact that they, like the unborn children, must make progress if they want to continue living.

OUT OF RESPECT

If the unborn child were able to discuss the topic of abortion with his mother, he would probably agree with her out of respect for her.

A BREAKDOWN IN COMMUNICATION

Abortion is, in some way, a breakdown in communication between the mother and the child in her womb.

A VICTIM OF POLITICS

Without voice and vote, the unborn child has no representation before government powers.

THE MAKING OF A MARTYR

A pregnant mother should know that by resorting to abortion, she turns her unborn child into a martyr.

CHAPTER III

LEGALIZED ABORTION

A DISCRIMINATORY LAW

The law institutionalizing abortion may protect the interests of a pregnant woman but denies those of the child in her womb.

ADVOCATES FOR ABORTION

The ill effects of abortion make a turn for the worst when the woman who has had an abortion chooses to become an advocate for abortion.

CONDITIONS FOR LEGALIZED ABORTION.

In order for a government to legalize abortion, three conditions are required, namely:

1. The inability or refusal of its socioeconomic system to meet the needs of the growing population.

2. A medical science sufficiently developed as to ensure the death of the unborn child while preserving the life of the mother.

3. A predominant collective believe that the unborn are not human.

INSTINCT OF SURVIVAL

Except for cases of extreme mental disorders that may lead to suicide, man always fights for survival. The human instinct for survival — like every human instinct – is formed in the womb. Abortion is the first and last defeat of the unborn child's survival instinct.

NO JUSTIFICATION

When there seems to be even one reason to justify abortion, that reason must be thoroughly examined with the eyes of human compassion, and it will be found that there is no such justification.

PARENTAL AWARENESS

The law regulates the external behavior of people, not their conscience. Thus, the issue of abortion will not be corrected by the law, but by the conscious awareness of the parents that abortion is the killing of the unborn child.

THE INABILITY OF AN ECONOMIC SYSTEM

When a woman feels that she is forced to abort her child because the economic system will not allow her to provide for the physical needs of her child, such an economic system should be overthrown due to its inability to provide for the most basic of all human needs.

THANKSGIVING

The first act of thanksgiving of those who are alive is that which we owe to our mother who did not abort us while we were in her womb.

———

ABORTION HARMS THE MOTHER

Abortion harms the human integrity of the mother, for when a society permits a mother to end the life of her unborn child through abortion, how can she be expected to respect the life of other human beings – including that of other unborn children?

———

NO EXPECTATION

Once abortion is legalized, there can be no expectation that the law will protect life at any stage of human development.

———

VIRTUE AND VICE

Power is a virtue the pregnant woman turns into a vice when she chooses abortion.

———

LIFE EXPECTANCY

Under legalized abortion, the life expectancy of an unborn child does not depend on the medical science; it depends on the law.

———

INEVITABLE DISCRIMINATION

When a society discriminates against the poor in favor of the rich, and against the weak in favor of the powerful, it is only a matter of time that the law will discriminate against the unborn in favor of those who have already been born.

———

A MATTER OF CONSCIENCE
When the law shows no respect for the life of the unborn, conscience must prevail over the law.

———————

A TRUE HEROINE
In times of legalized abortion, the woman who brings her pregnancy to completion is a true heroine.

———————

THE ISSUE OF KILLING.
Legalized abortion pretends to remove the issue of killing from the realm of the human conscience.

———————

LEGALIZATION
Legalized abortion means that the law has taken upon itself the prerogative to forgive sins by legalizing them.

———————

NOT A NIGHTTIME STORY FOR CHILDREN
Legalized abortion has turned the unborn child into a "little red riding hood", although with the variation that the wolf is her own mother.

———————

CHOICE IS FINE
Choice is fine. The issue is what you choose.

———————

CHOOSING LIFE

Humanity has been able to survive up to this point because it has chosen life over death.

THE CREED OF THE ABORTIONIST AND THE XENO-PHOBIC.

We believe that the immigrant and the unborn
have never done us any good,
they always have been known
for taking our jobs, our money, and our food.

A POWERFUL ALLY

Life loses a powerful ally with every woman that moves to the side of abortion.

SELF-DISQUALIFICATION

The abortionists have splendidly succeeded at taking themselves out of the human struggle for peace, justice, and life.

A GREAT LOSS

If the millions of children that have fallen to abortion had been born, it is certain that by now, we would have great scientists working on a cure for cancer, great economists, sociologists, and educators helping us to eradicate abortion.

THE VOICE OF LEGALIZED ABORTION

The law authorizing abortion solemnly proclaims: "To you all pregnant women of the world, you are the last line of defense for your unborn children because I, the Law of the Land, want them dead".

TWO POINTS OF VIEW

The back-alley abortion is different than the hospital abortion – from the medical point of view, of course. But, from the human point of view, they are exactly the same: they both kill the unborn and the soul of everyone involved.

ATTACK TO THE HEART

Legalized abortion attacks the very heart of the medical profession: it encourages death over life.

OPTIONS

Life opens all options; abortion closes them all.

IT FITS THE DEFINITION

The killing of a human being is defined as a homicide when the following elements concur: Intentionality, premeditation, and execution. Those elements are present in abortion.

NOBLE SPIRIT

Legalized abortion gives the unborn child the opportunity to show his noble spirit: out of respect for his parents, he would not file murder charges against them.

A PRICE TO PAY

Once abortion is legalized, abortion becomes the price the unborn child pays for reminding his parents of their parental responsibilities.

IGNORANCE

Ignoring God leads to ignorance of Nature, and ignorance of Nature leads to all sorts of human aberrations.

A MEANS OF OPPRESSION

The law becomes a means of oppression when it denies the unborn child's right to be born.

GENOCIDAL POWERS

In a country where abortion is legal, the death of millions of unborn children is a denunciation of the genocidal powers of the law.

IT IS UP TO THE PARENTS

We know that "the law is for man, not man for the law". It is up to the parents of the unborn child to demonstrate that the law does not have the power to destroy life.

WHO SPEAKS LOUDER?

Procreation is the voice of life. Abortion is the voice of death. Legalized abortion indicates that death speaks louder than life.

EXCUSES

In order to legalize abortion, an ineffective economic system gives the following excuse: "there are too many mouths to feed."

NOT ONLY IN WAR

Abortion contradicts the notion that men systematically kill one another only in times of war.

THE GOD OF DEATH

There are a few religious groups that approved abortion. Those groups worship a god of death.

IT MUST BE STOPED

The elimination of unborn children by legalized abortion may last indefinitely, unless the parents say no to abortion.

A LETHAL WEAPON

Nobody ever thought that the most lethal weapon of mass destruction would be utilized in our health care facilities: abortion.

METAMORPHOSIS.

Abortion is the metamorphosis of the primitive instinct to kill animals for the survival of our species into the habit of killing other human beings for the destruction of our species.

TRUE HEALING

The collective belief that abortion is not the killing of a human being will simply numb the conscience of the mother. True healing will come only when she makes the commitment not to have another abortion.

UNWORTHY OF LIVING

Legalized abortion is only feasible in a society that considers life unworthy of living, even the life of the mother.

SYSTEMATIC DESTRUCTION

Through millions of years of evolution man was able to elevate himself from the animal kingdom to the human kingdom. However, in recent times, through war and abortion, man is causing his own regression to levels below the animal kingdom. For no animal species is known to cause its own systematic destruction.

PREYING ON HIMSELF

Abortion, like war, turns a human being into a formidable animal of prey, preying on its own species.

ONLY THE PARENTS CAN DO IT

A decision by the United States Supreme Court to repeal abortion will not be sufficient to end abortion. Only the parents' decision will.

NO SELF-DEFENSE

The benefit of self-defense cannot be invoked in favor of those who resort to abortion or in favor of the society that legalizes it.

IT'S BEEN FOUND

Finally, some nations have found a way to kill human beings without considering it a crime: kill them before they are born!

CHANGING TIMES

Since the human race appeared on the face of the earth, parents have protected their children, but nowadays they have the choice to kill them through abortion.

UNKNOWN ABORTION

All species of animals protect their offspring. They don't know about abortion.

EVEN IF...

Even if there were nothing divine in human life, abortion would still be responsible for taking even the humanness out of human life.

THE VOICE OF CREATION

Life is the voice of creation inside and outside a person. Abortion silences the voice of creation.

BIRTH AND BURIAL

The birth of a child is the most exultant expression of man's creative power. Abortion is the burial of such creative power and of man himself.

———

SPREADING CANCER

Once the cancerous cells of abortion appear in the organism of humanity, it is only a matter of time before the cancer spreads to the cells of justice, peace, and all other healthy cells of humanity's organism.

———

A GOOD REASON

Abortion is not abominable because God prohibits it; God prohibits it because abortion is abominable.

———

BE CAREFUL WITH WHAT YOU PRAY FOR

To those who pray for an end to abortion, God gives them life. And to those who pray for the continuation of abortion, God gives them life, as well. But the latter swear not to ask God for anything again.

———

NEGATION PLUS

Science shows that life before birth and life after birth are full of wonderful achievements. Abortion not only negates the achievements in both stages of life but it also sinks humankind in darkness.

———

IRREVOCABLE SENTENCE

No matter how many times the unborn child may plead his innocence, no matter how much he may prove his rehabilitation, no matter how much he may show good conduct, all is irrelevant. The parents have already testified that they do not want him. Therefore, pursuant to the law legalizing abortion, the unborn child is sentenced to death by abortion.

ABORTING THE TRUTH

Some people believe they have succeeded in justifying abortion. But, in fact, they have only succeeded in aborting the truth.

FOR STARTERS

A society, which looks for justifications to kill the elderly, starts by killing the unborn.

NO REASON TO EXIST

The ultimate reason for the existence of the State is the protection of the life of its citizens. By legalizing abortion, the State has lost the reason for its existence.

SEXUAL CONTROL

If men and women had control over their sexual impulses, as it is expected of human beings, there would be no abortion.

IT IS NOT FREEDOM

To believe that abortion is an expression of freedom will lead us to believe that harming unborn children is also an expression of freedom.

WHEN AUTHORITY MUST BE TAKEN AWAY

When the State grants the parents the right to terminate the life of their unborn child because he is considered to be a liability to them, the State must be stripped of its authority to impose laws on its citizens.

DOUBLE DENIAL

Every human being has a right to a future. Legalized abortion denies that right not only to the unborn child but also to the entire humanity.

ENDING WITH THE FIRST

If abortion were an element of human nature, the human race would not have survived past the first couple.

THINK TWICE

It is not rare for an elderly person to say he wishes to be young again. And why not as young as a child who is in his mother's womb? But in a world where abortion is legal, the elderly person might have to think twice.

ALLEGING IGNORANCE

It is a principle of criminal law that ignorance of certain facts may exonerate the perpetrator from guilt, as long as said ignorance is not intentional. When confronted with the charges of murder, the author of the abortion law has pleaded "not guilty" on the grounds he is ignorant of the fact that human life begins at conception. But in this case, the benefit of ignorance is not applicable because the author of the law is intentionally ignorant.

IN THE DARKNESS

In the darkness of twilight, a hunter kills a man thinking he is a deer. In the darkness of society, those who legalized abortion kill millions of unborn children, thinking they are not human.

SILENT LAMBS

The victims of abortion march to their death like silent lambs to the slaughterhouse.

OVERPOPULATION OF ANGELS

Since abortion was legalized on earth, heaven is having an overpopulation of little angels.

UNDENIABLE PROOF

When the aborted children arrive in heaven, God sees them as the proof that humanity is in decadence.

NO LAWS

Legalized abortion is one of the reasons why the primitive human community did not have any laws.

SECRET ABORTION

The parents who, after having had several children, abort their youngest child, may need to keep that abortion secret in order to prevent the older children from questioning their parents' commitment to them.

AGAINST QUALITY OF LIFE

The killing of unborn children, as a means to reduce population growth, will only reduce the quality of life for every living person.

AN OUTRAGEOUS LOGIC

When an enemy threatens the interests of a nation, that nation may proceed to destroy its enemy. When an unborn child threatens the interests of his parents, the latter may proceed to abort the former.

ANIMALS DON'T KNOW ABOUT ABORTION

The perpetuation of the species is the reason why animals do not kill their offspring; humans add another reason: respect for life. That is why abortion renders human beings inferior to animals.

UNWORTHY OF LIVING

The parents who decide to abort their child, consider their own image and likeness to be ugly and unworthy of living.

———————

LEGALIZED ABORTION AND DECLARED WAR

Legalized abortion means the killing of the unborn child with the approval of the law. Declaring war means the killing of the enemy with the approval of the law.

———————

MOURNING FOR SOCIETY

The aborted child mourns, not so much for his own death but for the moral death of the society that approves abortion.

———————

FOR COSMETIC REASONS

Abortion for cosmetic reasons may lead a woman to believe that her body will remain beautiful, but not her soul.

———————

STARVATION

When we recommend abortion in order to avoid feeding another mouth, we recommend the starvation of the human race.

———————

WE CAN NEVER HAVE ENOUGH...

If we agree that we can never have enough of a good thing, then those who believe that abortion is a good thing must also believe that the extinction of the human race is a good thing.

———————

FEWER NEIGHBORS

Since love of neighbor is becoming increasingly more difficult, some people are resorting to any possible means to reduce the number of their neighbors. One of those means is abortion.

———————

UNITED

War and abortion are twin brothers united by the killing of human beings.

———————

MISERY LOVES COMPANY

Most of those who, at one time or another, had an abortion or were involved in an abortion, become advocates for abortion because they believe that the larger the number of abortions, the lesser the guilt.

———————

AN INCONVENIENCE

Under legalized abortion, the unborn child is killed not because he is bad or good, ugly or cute, rich or poor, but because he is an inconvenience to his parents, to society, or to both.

———————

EVERYBODY'S ISSUE

Abortion is a mother's issue. However, when there is a mother, there is a father; and no one is a mother or a father unless there is a child. But since mother, father, or child cannot exist without society, we have to conclude that abortion is everybody's issue.

———————

DEFENSELESS

The easiest way to kill a human being is abortion. The unborn child is totally defenseless.

VIOLENCE FROM THE LAW

The fact that the law approves abortion is an indication that there is such thing as legal violence.

UTTERLY DISTURBING

One of the most disturbing aspects of abortion is that while Mother Nature wants the unborn child to be born, his biological parents want him to die.

DOUBLE HARM

Abortion not only harms the life of an individual; it also harms the integrity of the collectivity.

SLAVERY AND ABORTION

Just as slavery is the negation of liberty, abortion is the negation of life.

ANXIETY

There was a time when the unborn child lived happily in his mother's womb. But when abortion is legal, he lives in a constant state of anxiety.

THE SAME FIGHT

The fight against abortion is part of the fight against social injustice.

THE FIGHT FOR SOCIAL JUSTICE

He who fights for social justice must fight for life and for the integrity of the family.

COST EFFECTIVE

A nation that legalizes abortion has one objective in mind: to prove that it is cost effective to reduce the population by getting rid of the most defenseless of all human beings, even before they set foot on earth.

NO JURISDICTION

Legalized abortion takes away the jurisdiction of the courts to hear crimes against life.

WEAKNESS AND IGNORANCE

Abortion is always a sign of weakness, for it proves that neither parents nor society are strong enough to defend the unborn child. And, if the ensuing question is, what is there to defend" Then, abortion is also a sign of a grave ignorance on the part of parents and society.

GOOD LUCK TO YOU

Where abortion is legalized, the newly conceived child hopes for good luck because he needs it more than the adults.

A WOMAN'S MANIFESTO

All pregnant women of the world, unite! Abortion is the worse form of exploitation of a human being by another human being.

AUTHORIZATION AND REVOCATION

The law may authorize abortion; the mother may revoke it.

DEPRESSION

Any proposal for the legalization of abortion is enough to plant the seeds of depression in the unborn child.

SUICIDE

Abortion is the means humanity chooses to commit suicide.

NO FOOD, NO LIFE

Abortion consists in depriving the unborn child of the life he needs to be born, just as starvation consists in depriving an adult person of the food he needs to continue living.

A TRAGIC VICTORY

The parents of the newly conceived child know it is true that they have created a new human being. Legalized abortion is the victory of the lie over the truth.

DESTROYER OF TREASURES

The unborn child has only two treasures: life and the love of his parents. Abortion destroys both.

———

WHY SHOULD HE PAY FOR OTHERS' FAILURES?

Some people may say that a pregnant woman, abandoned by relatives and friends, accused of adultery, homeless, unemployed, with no money, without medical care has a right to have an abortion. The question is: Why does the unborn child have to pay, with his life, for the failures of a society we adults are unwilling to correct?

———

NO RIGHT TO APPEAL

Legalized abortion deprives the unborn child not only of the right to life but also of the right to appeal a death sentence.

———

WHEN THE REMEDY KILLS

In a society where the conflicts between men are resolved by mutual destruction, the conflicts between the mother and her unborn child are resolved by legalized abortion.

———

DISCRIMINATORY PREMISE

Legalized abortion is predicated on the premise that there are some children who do not deserve to be born.

———

THE THREAT OF LEGALIZED ABORTION

With the threat of legalized abortion pending over his head, the unborn child must live each day as if it were his last.

CONFISCATION AND LEGALIZED ABORTION

Just as the State has the power to authorize a person to take another person's possessions in accordance with legalized confiscation, so too does it have the power to authorize a mother to take her unborn child's life in accordance with legalized abortion.

WHO IS A FAILURE?

The unborn child is not a failure on account of legalized abortion, society is.

A HELLISH ALLIANCE

When abortion is legalized, the unborn child has to contend against a hellish alliance: the State and its underlings.

FEMINIST PROTECTION

Feminists must be against abortion because they have to protect the life of an unborn female child.

FEMINISM AND ABORTION ARE INCOMPATIBLE

Feminism is based on equal rights for men and women. Abortion is based on unequal rights for women and their unborn children.

RUSSIAN ROULETTE

Abortion is like a game of Russian roulette whereby the law gives a pregnant mother a revolver loaded with only one bullet for her to hold, not against her head, but against the head of her unborn child.

———————

RESEMBLANCE

There is nothing that resembles a war of aggression more than abortion, with the parents being the aggressors.

———————

SURVIVORS

In any natural disaster, the likelihood of finding survivors is quite real, but in the human disaster of abortion, the likelihood of survivors is zero.

———————

GREAT IGNORANCE

Abortion is possible only when the parents choose to ignore the fact that the child in the mother's womb is a human being.

———————

THE WAY WE WERE

If you are in favor of abortion now, remember that, at one time in the past, you were an embryo.

———————

A PERVERTED WORLD

We live in a perverted world because men have been given the right to kill their enemies, and pregnant mothers have been given the right to abort their children.

FOR WHOM CAN THEY MOURN?

If humans lack the sensitivity to mourn for an aborted child, for whom can they mourn?

THE RIGHT TO PROCREATE

Abortion is an infringement on the pregnant woman's right to bring forth life.

TWO ABORTIONS

The abortion of a child occurs when society aborts its responsibility to protect the life of the unborn.

CANNOT REJOICE

Whenever society and the pregnant mother cannot rejoice at the presence of a newly conceived child, abortion becomes an option.

A MYSTERY SOLVED

A historical analysis of legalized abortion may shed light upon the possibility that the dinosaurs became extinct after they began to step on each other's eggs.

TWO OPPOSING VOICES

When it comes to legalized abortion, Mother Nature speaks up for the protection of life, whereas, the State speaks up for the termination of life.

———————

"THEY DON'T GIVE A DAMN"

Some so-called "professionals" advise a poor pregnant mother to abort her unborn child so that she may have a better life and that her child may not suffer a life of unhappiness. The mother should know, however, that these "professionals" truly don't give a damn about the mother or the child.

———————

ILL-ADVISED

To recommend abortion, in order to prevent the birth of a poor child, is equivalent to recommending the killing of the poor in order to end poverty.

———————

COMPLYING WITH JUSTICE

In order to comply with justice, the law must protect the life of the pregnant mother and the life of the unborn.

———————

DECISIONS, DECISIONS

The problem with abortion is that the pregnant mother does not decide about her life but about someone else's life.

———————

REPRODUCTIVE RIGHTS

How can a woman claim reproductive rights if, by resorting to abortion, she brings reproduction to an end?

———————

A LEGAL FARCE

When the law fails to protect the life of the pregnant mother and the life of the unborn, we are dealing with a legal farce.

———

IN THE HEART OF THE MATTER

The core of abortion rights: have sexual intercourse anytime and resort to abortion on demand.

———

TERMINAL ILLNESS

Abortion is a terminal illness to the unborn.

———

WHAT CAN WE DO?

The judicial authorization, the legislative accord, and the medical intervention to facilitate the performance of a single abortion renders the judge, the legislator, and the physician guilty of terminating a life and conspiracy to terminate a life. And as for the rest of us, it all depends on what we do.

———

DATA ABOUT ABORTION IN THE U.S.

(Exerts from the study "What the data says about abortion in the U.S." prepared by Jeff Diamant and Besheer Mohamed and published through the Internet on June 22, 2022 by the Pew Research Center).

Pew Research Center has conducted many surveys about abortion over the years, providing a lens into Americans' views on whether the procedure should be legal, among a host of other questions. In our most recent survey, 61% of U.S. adults say abortion should be legal all or most of the time, while 37% say it should be illegal all or most of the time.

With the U.S. Supreme Court's decision in Dobbs v. Jackson Women's Health Organization overturning Roe v. Wade, the 1973 case that effectively legalized abortion nationwide, here is a look at the most recent available data about abortion from sources other than public opinion surveys.

How many abortions are there in the United States each year?

An exact answer is hard to come by. Two organizations – the Centers for Disease Control and Prevention (CDC) and the Guttmacher Institute – try to measure this, but they use different methods and publish different figures.

The CDC compiles figures voluntarily reported by the central health agencies of the vast majority of states (including separate figures for New York City) and the District of Columbia. Its latest totals do not include figures from California, Maryland or New Hampshire, which did not report data to the CDC.

The Guttmacher Institute compiles its figures after contacting every known provider of abortions – clinics, hospitals and physicians' offices – in the country. It uses questionnaires and health department data, and it provides estimates for abortion providers that don't respond to its inquiries. In part because Guttmacher includes figures (and in some instances, estimates) from all 50 states, its totals are higher than the CDC's.

The last year for which the CDC reported a yearly national total for abortions is 2019. The agency says there were 629,898 abortions nationally that year, slightly up from 619,591 in 2018. Guttmacher's latest available figures are from 2020, when it says there were 930,160 abortions nationwide, up from 916,460 in 2019.

It's worth noting that the figures reported by both organizations include only the legal induced abortions conducted by clinics, hospitals or physicians' offices, or that make use of abortion pills dispensed from certified facilities such as clinics or physicians' offices. They do not account for the use of abortion pills that were obtained outside of clinical settings.

How has the number of abortions in the U.S. changed over the years?
The following years are selected from the report published by the Guttmacher Institute:
- In 1973 --------------- 774,000 abortions.
- In 1990 -------------- 1'600,000 abortions.
- In 1996 -------------- 1'200,000 abortions.
- In 2020 ------------- 930,160 abortions.

The annual number of U.S. abortions rose for years after Roe v. Wade legalized the procedure in 1973, reaching its highest levels around the late 1980s and early 1990s, according to both the CDC and

Guttmacher. Since then, it has generally decreased at what a CDC analysis called "a slow yet steady pace."

There have been occasional breaks in this long-term pattern of decline – during the middle of the first decade of the 2000s, and then again in the late 2010s. The CDC reported modest 1% and 2% increases in abortions in 2018 and 2019, respectively, while Guttmacher reported an 8% increase in abortions over the three-year period from 2017 to 2020.

As noted above, these figures do not include abortions that use pills that were obtained outside of clinical settings.

What is the abortion rate among women in the U.S.?
How has it changed over time?

Guttmacher says that in 2020 there were 14.4 abortions in the U.S. per 1,000 women ages 15 to 44. Its data shows that the rate of abortions among women has generally been declining in the U.S. since 1981, when it reported there were 29.3 abortions per 1,000 women in that age range.

The CDC says that in 2019, there were 11.4 abortions in the U.S. per 1,000 women ages 15 to 44. (That figure excludes California, Maryland, New Hampshire and the District of Columbia.) Like Guttmacher's data, the CDC's figures also suggest a general decline in the abortion rate over time. In 1980, when the CDC reported on all 50 states and D.C., it said there were 25 abortions per 1,000 women ages 15 to 44.

That said, both Guttmacher and the CDC say there were slight increases in the rate of abortions during the late 2010s. Guttmacher says the abortion rate per 1,000 women ages 15 to 44 rose from 13.5 in 2017 to 14.4 in 2020. The CDC says it rose from 11.2 in 2017 to 11.4 in 2019. (The CDC's figures for both of those years exclude data from California, Maryland, New Hampshire and the District of Columbia).

What are the most common types of abortion?

The CDC broadly divides abortions into two categories: surgical abortions and medication abortions. In 2019, 56% of legal abortions in clinical settings occurred via some form of surgery, while 44% were medication abortions involving pills, according to the CDC. Since the Food and Drug Administration first approved abortion pills in 2000, their use has increased over time as a share of abortions nationally. Guttmacher's preliminary data from its forthcoming study says that 2020 was the first time that more than half of all abortions in clinical settings in the U.S. were medication abortions.

Two pills commonly used together for medication abortions are mifepristone, which, taken first, blocks hormones that support a pregnancy, and misoprostol, which then causes the uterus to empty. Medication abortion is approved for use until 10 weeks into pregnancy.

Surgical abortions conducted during the first trimester of pregnancy typically use a suction process, while the relatively few surgical abortions that occur during the second trimester of a pregnancy typically use a process called dilation and evacuation, according to the UCLA School of Medicine website.

How many abortion providers are there in the U.S., and how has that number changed over time?

In 2017, there were 1,587 facilities in the U.S. that provided abortions, according to Guttmacher. This included 808 clinics, 518 hospitals and 261 physicians' offices.

While clinics make up a slight majority (51%) of the facilities that provide abortions, they are the sites where the vast majority (95%) of abortions occur, including 60% at specialized abortion clinics and 35% at nonspecialized clinics, according to the 2017 data from Guttmacher. Hospitals made up 33% of the facilities that provided abortions but accounted for only 3% of abortions that year, while just 1% of abortions were conducted by physicians' offices.

Looking just at clinics – that is, the total number of specialized abortion clinics and nonspecialized clinics in the U.S. – Guttmacher found a 2% increase between 2014 and 2017. However, there were regional differences. In the Northeast, the number of clinics that provide abortions increased by 16% during those years, and in the West by 4%. The number of clinics decreased during those years by 9% in the South and 6% in the Midwest.

The total number of abortion providers has declined dramatically since the 1980s. In 1982, according to Guttmacher, there were 2,908 facilities providing abortions in the U.S., including 789 clinics, 1,405 hospitals and 714 physicians' offices.

Later this year, Guttmacher is expected to publish a similar breakdown of the types of abortion providers for 2020. The CDC does not track the number of abortion providers.

What percentage of abortions are for women who live in a different state from the abortion provider?

In the District of Columbia, New York City and the 47 states that provided information to the CDC in 2019, 9.3% of all abortions were performed on women whose state of residency was known to be different than the state where the abortion occurred – virtually the same percentage as in the previous year.

The share of reported abortions performed on women outside their state of residence was much higher before the 1973 Roe decision that stopped states from banning abortion. In 1972, 41% of all abortions in D.C. or the 20 states that provided this information to the CDC that year were performed on women outside their state of residence. In 1973, the corresponding figure was 21% in D.C. and the 41 states that provided this information, and in 1974 it was 11% in D.C. and the 43 states that provided data.

Anticipating that many states will further restrict abortion access, politicians in some states with permissive abortion laws such as New York, California and Oregon are expecting more women from states with less abortion access to travel to their states for an abortion.

What are the demographics of women who had abortions in 2019?

In the District of Columbia and 47 states that reported data to the CDC in 2019, the majority of women who had abortions (57%) were in their 20s, while about three-in-ten (31%) were in their 30s. Teens ages 13 to 19 accounted for 9% of those who had abortions, while women in their 40s accounted for 4%.

The vast majority of women who had abortions in 2019 were un-married (85%), while married women accounted for 15%, according to the CDC, which had data on this from 41 states and New York City (but not the rest of New York).

In the District of Columbia and 29 states that reported racial and ethnic data on abortion to the CDC, 38% of all women who had abor-tions in 2019 were non-Hispanic Black, while 33% were non-Hispanic White, 21% were Hispanic, and 7% were of other races or ethnicities.

Among those ages 15 to 44, there were 23.8 abortions per 1,000 non-Hispanic Black women; 11.7 abortions per 1,000 Hispanic women; 6.6 abortions per 1,000 non-Hispanic White women; and 13 abortions per 1,000 women of other races or ethnicities in that age range, the CDC reported from those same 29 states and the District of Columbia.

For 58% of U.S. women who had induced abortions in 2019, it was the first time they had ever had one, according to the CDC. For nearly a quarter (24%), it was their second abortion. For 11% of women, it was their third, and for 8% it was their fourth or higher. These CDC figures include data from 43 states and New York City (but not the rest of New York).

In 2019, most U.S. abortions were for women who had already given birth.

Four-in-ten women who had abortions in 2019 (40%) had no pre-vious live births at the time they had an abortion, according to the CDC. A quarter of women (25%) who had abortions in 2019 had one previous live birth, 20% had two previous live births, 9% had three, and 6% had four or more previous live births. These CDC figures include data from 44 states and New York City (but not the rest of New York).

When during pregnancy do most abortions occur?

The vast majority of abortions – around nine-in-ten – occur during the first trimester of a pregnancy. In 2019, 93% of abortions occurred during the first trimester – that is, at or before 13 weeks of gestation, according to the CDC. An additional 6% occurred between 14 and 20 weeks of pregnancy, and 1% were performed at 21 weeks or more of gestation. These CDC figures include data from 42 states and New York City (but not the rest of New York).

How often are there medical complications from abortion?

About 2% of all abortions in the U.S. involve some type of complication for the woman, according to the National Center for Biotechnology Information, which is part of the U.S. National Library of Medicine, a branch of the National Institutes of Health. The center says that "most complications are considered minor such as pain, bleeding, infection and post-anesthesia complications."

The CDC calculates case-fatality rates for women from legal induced abortions – that is, how many women die from complications from abortion, for every 100,000 abortions that occur in the U.S. The rate was lowest during the most recent period examined by the agency (2013 to 2018), when there were 0.4 deaths to women per 100,000 legal induced abortions. The case-fatality rate reported by the CDC was highest during the first period examined by the agency (1973 to 1977), when it was 2.1 deaths to women per 100,000 legal induced abortions.

During the five-year periods in between, the figure ranged from 0.5 (from 1993 to 1997) to 0.8 (from 1978 to 1982). The CDC says it calculates death rates by five-year and six-year periods because of year-to-year fluctuation in the numbers and due to the relatively low number of women who die from abortion.

Two women died from induced abortion in the U.S. in 2018, in both cases from abortions that were legal, according to the CDC. The same was true in 2017. In 2016, the CDC reported seven deaths from either legal (six) or illegal (one) induced abortions. Since 1990, the annual number of deaths among women due to induced abortion has ranged from two to 12, according to the CDC.

The annual number of reported deaths from induced abortions tended to be higher in the 1980s, when it ranged from nine to 16, and from 1972 to 1979, when it ranged from 13 to 54 (1972 was the first year the CDC began collecting this data). One driver of the decline was the drop in deaths from illegal abortions. There were 35 deaths from illegal abortions in 1972, the last full year before Roe v. Wade.

The total fell to 19 in 1973 and to single digits or zero every year after that. (The number of deaths from legal abortions has also declined since then, though with some slight variation over time.)

The number of deaths from induced abortions was considerably higher in the 1960s than afterward. For instance, there were 235 deaths from abortions in 1965 and 280 in 1963, according to reports by the then-U.S. Department of Health, Education and Welfare, a precursor to the Department of Health and Human Services. The CDC is a division of Health and Human Services.

www.ingramcontent.com/pod-product-compliance
Lightning Source LLC
Chambersburg PA
CBHW060753260726
48660CB00002B/608